Overcoming

Postpartum Depression

with Resilience

Caring for baby, Caring for you

Dr. Monica Haman

Other Books by This Author

https://www.amazon.com/dp/B0BT9912YX

https://www.amazon.com/dp/B0BX2FRN1Q

https://www.amazon.com/dp/B0BRX25GC6

https://www.amazon.com/dp/B0BSTMZ7PJ

https://www.amazon.com/dp/B0BRDGMMRB

https://www.amazon.com/dp/B0BRDGMMRB

https://www.amazon.com/dp/B0CMPMCG97

https://www.amazon.com/dp/B0CN7FPYJG

TABLE OF CONTENTS

INTRODUCTION

When I discovered I was going to be a mom, I had this whole script in my head—a seamless blend of maternal instinct, unconditional love, and a picturesque journey into motherhood. But here's the unfiltered truth: reality hits harder than a ton of bricks. Labour was not the emotional crescendo I expected; instead, it felt like I'd run a marathon with no finish line, and the only sentiment that prevailed was relief, mingled with an overwhelming exhaustion that no amount of sleep could ease.

In the days and weeks that followed, the dreams of being a flawless mom crumbled. Love at first sight? More like a vague sense of responsibility, lacking the warmth I'd anticipated. It was disorienting, and I felt like I'd failed—not just as a mom, but also as a doctor who, by all accounts, should have had it figured out.

This book isn't a glossy facade of perfect motherhood. It's a gritty, real account of the emotional labyrinth that is postpartum life. I'm not here to sugarcoat; I'm here to share how it felt to grapple with that double sense of failure—failing my expectations as a mom and grappling with the haunting notion that, as a doctor, I should have been immune to this.

In those vulnerable weeks, I wasn't a poster mom; I was just a woman navigating the unexpected terrain of motherhood. I want you to know that if you've ever felt like you're not measuring up to the societal notion of the perfect mom, you're not alone. These postpartum struggles aren't anomalies; they're more common than we care to admit.

As a fellow mom and a doctor who thought she had all the answers, I get it. I get the silent battles, the feeling of questioning your worth, and the persistent notion that you're not living up to your own expectations, let alone society's. But here's where the narrative shifts. This isn't just a memoir of struggles; it's a guide, a beacon of assurance, and a testament that even in the darkest corners of motherhood, resilience can bloom.

This book isn't just a collection of words; it's a lifeline that helped me navigate through the shadows and rediscover the joy in being a mom. I share practices, insights, and real-life moments that became stepping stones back to the light. It's not a promise to have all the answers, but it's a pledge to share what I've learned in the hope that it might ease your journey.

So, as we embark on this exploration of postpartum challenges, let's cast away the façade of perfection and embrace the messy, beautiful reality of being a mom. This isn't a guide from someone who's got it all figured out;

it's a companionate narrative from a fellow traveller who understands the double sense of failure and emerged stronger on the other side. I invite you to join me, not as an authority but as a friend who's been there, felt that, and come out the other side with insights worth sharing.

Chapter One

Understanding Postpartum Depression

We are often bombarded with expectations of instant joy and an unshakable link with our child in the silent moments following bringing a new life into the world.

For some of us, however, the truth is far more nuanced, and it is essential to recognize this. Together, let's learn about the complexities of postpartum depression and provide a welcoming environment for new mothers who are struggling with feelings they didn't know they were capable of experiencing.

Experiencing postpartum depression does not render a mother less capable of caring for her child. It doesn't discriminate, whether this is your first journey into motherhood or whether you're a seasoned parent.

It can develop in ways you don't expect, creeping in subtly when you thought your life could only get better. It is necessary to dispel the myth that mothers experiencing postpartum depression are inadequate workers.

In popular culture, mothers and their newborns are depicted as sharing an instant bond from the moment the baby takes its first breath. But the real world is more complicated and messy. It's quite normal if you don't feel an overwhelming surge of feeling right away.

In the first few hours, days, or weeks, it's normal to feel a range of emotions you haven't experienced before.

The onset and duration of postpartum depression are arbitrary. Hormonal fluctuations, environmental stressors, and a mother's individual life experiences all play a role in this process. It's a haze that might make it hard to see past the happy moment of giving birth.

In reality, postpartum melancholy extends much beyond the initial "baby blues." It's a clinical disorder that goes beyond the normal emotional ups and downs experienced by many new mothers. It includes emotions like melancholy, anxiety, and a generalised sense of worthlessness that last for weeks, months, or even years.

It's important to keep in mind that postpartum depression obscures the lens through which you see your child's love, not diminishes it. This chapter serves as a gentle reminder that the journey to parenthood is diverse, and the emotions that accompany it are similarly unique.

The path of motherhood, like any other journey, is not without its difficulties. It's normal for your bond with your newborn to develop gradually. The connection between a mother and her kid develops gradually over time, rather than appearing fully formed all at once.

Let's take an attitude of compassion as we negotiate the challenging terrain of postpartum depression. Realising that you are not alone on your journey, that your feelings are understandable, and that reaching out for assistance is not a show of weakness but a brave step towards recovery.

In the following chapters, we'll go more into the effects of postpartum depression, the power of resilience, and the importance of surrounding yourself with positive people to help you heal.

Chapter Two

The Impact of Postpartum Depression

Understanding the complex nature of postpartum depression is crucial because of the far-reaching effects it can have on a mother's daily life. This section examines the secondary impacts of postpartum depression, recognizing that it has far-reaching implications for the mother's and child's health beyond the realm of emotions alone.

Emotional Well-Being

Postpartum depression is characterised by tangled feelings of despair, worry, and complete lack of self-worth. The emotional cost is not something you feel once and then forget about; rather, it hangs over the happy, bonding times with your newborn. In order to create successful techniques for coping and healing, it is essential to have a thorough understanding of the complexities of this emotional environment.

Strain on Relationships

Postpartum depression can have an impact on friendships, family, and partnerships. The difficulty of helping a loved one through this maze of feelings can put a strain on even the strongest of bonds.

The stresses that postpartum depression can cause in interpersonal connections are examined, and suggestions on how to provide the understanding and compassion that are so vital at this time are provided.

Daily Functioning and Parenting

Managing the rigours of everyday life becomes difficult for moms who are experiencing postpartum depression. What was once a breeze becomes an enormous obstacle. The pleasant responsibilities of parenthood may be eclipsed by a pervading sense of exhaustion and despondency.

When I woke up to my crying newborn, that was the precise time that I felt the full effect of postpartum depression's physical and mental load.

I can still remember the exact moment very clearly. The difficulty I had in calming my sobbing child was indicative of the extent to which this had an effect on my ability to operate normally and raise my children.

The basic act of consoling my newborn seemed unachievable as I lay there, unable to move a muscle. It is a common issue for many mothers dealing with postpartum depression. It's during these exposed moments that the significant influence on day-to-day operations is most noticeable.

The Impact on the Child

Most importantly, the early experiences and development of the kid are negatively impacted by postpartum depression. The mother's emotional health and the child's feeling of safety and comfort are closely related. Comprehending this influence is the first step towards developing a comprehensive recovery strategy—realising that attending to the mother's health is essential to creating a loving atmosphere for the kid.

In this in-depth investigation, we address the complex effects of postpartum depression with compassion and useful knowledge. By recognizing its pervasiveness throughout a new mother's life, we open the door to all-encompassing solutions and durable avenues for recovery.

Let's work together to traverse these intricacies and cultivate an understanding that is essential to a transformative healing process.

Chapter Three

The Significance of Resilience in

Surmounting Postpartum Depression

Amidst the darkness and turmoil of postpartum depression, there is a glimmer of hope: resilience. The transforming force of resilience is explored in depth in this chapter, revealing its important role in overcoming the difficulties associated with postpartum depression.

Understanding Resilience

Every mother has the strength of character to endure adversity and come out on the other side stronger because of it. Understanding that resilience is not invulnerability but rather the activation of inner power in the face of adversity is vital.

Understanding resilience in the context of postpartum depression is like unearthing a latent superpower, one that equips us to confront the shadows and emerge into the light of recovery.

The Ebb and Flow of Postpartum Depression

Recognizing that periods of vulnerability are not setbacks but significant aspects of the journey is essential. Having the ability to bounce back quickly from setbacks is crucial during the healing process, which is fraught with complexity and uncertainty. These low points are when the tide of resilience rises and carries us over the difficulties.

The Unique Strength Every Mother Possesses

What makes every mother special: Each woman brings a distinct power to the dance of parenting, one that is perfectly tuned to her kid.

This strength from inside provides a solid foundation for bouncing back. Understanding the subtleties of a baby's cries, having an innate sense of what they need, and being steadfast in your determination to meet those needs are all part of this.

Let's honour the unique fortitude of every mother and recognize it as a source of tremendous fortitude

in the face of postpartum depression as we continue
to study resilience.

The Role of Professional Support

Having the guidance of experts who are familiar
with the landscape is crucial to building resilience.
In this piece, we'll look at how therapists,
counsellors, and other healthcare professionals can
help build resilience in their patients.

Their advice is a reliable map for mothers dealing
with postpartum depression, and they do so with
knowledge and empathy.

Any progress made while suffering from
postpartum depression is cause for celebration. This
chapter emphasises the necessity of recognizing
minor victories—whether it's a day of improved

mood or a moment of connection with your child. The hope that healing is not only attainable but a lifelong path is strengthened by these commemorations.

Chapter Four

Recognizing the Signs and Symptoms of

Postpartum Depression

Postpartum depression (PPD) is a prevalent disorder affecting recently given birth women. Knowing the symptoms of postpartum depression (PPD) is the first step to seeking help, raising awareness, and initiating the recovery process.

It is helpful for new moms and their loved ones, as well as the medical professionals who care for them, to understand the wide range of mental and physical symptoms associated with postpartum depression.

Subtle Signals of an Internal Struggle

Social norms and expectations for a happy postpartum period can obscure the emotional toll of postpartum depression. Picture a new mom who manages to keep her composure for the camera even while she's experiencing a perfect storm of emotions.

The ups and downs of motherhood are transformed into an ever-present fog of melancholy by this emotional load. This internal conflict can be recognized by paying close attention to the mother's tone of voice, facial expressions, and general manner.

Physical Manifestations: Bodily Clues

There is no denying the physical tiredness that comes with giving delivery, but postpartum depression adds a whole other level. Imagine a mother who, despite getting enough sleep, is overcome with exhaustion that goes much beyond the typical weariness that comes with caring for a newborn.

Subtle but important signs can be gleaned from changes in hunger, whether they are abnormally high or low. The toll taken on one's body and psyche can be seen clearly in the form of sleep disruptions. To stop brushing these symptoms off as normal postpartum difficulties and start paying attention to your body again, you need to stop discounting them.

Cognitive and Behavioural Shifts

Postpartum depression emerges in disruptions within the cognitive and behavioural landscape of a new mother. Imagine a woman, previously focused and resolute, now suffering with intrusive thoughts, persistent remorse, and an inexplicable sense of inadequacy.

The priorities have shifted when even the smallest activities become impossible. This internal conflict is a symptom of postpartum depression, which alters a mother's way of thinking and behaving in the world.

The Importance of Self-Reflection

Understanding the warning signals of PPD requires serious introspection. Imagine a mother writing in a journal, delving into the nuances of her feelings and taking stock of how her physical and mental health have evolved. Intentional self-awareness acts as a candle, shedding light on previously hidden aspects of one's character. Taking part in these activities can help a mother understand her own mental health better and be better prepared to spot the minor signs of postpartum depression.

The Role of Loved Ones: Supporting Recognition

Acknowledging something takes the love and understanding of others; it is not a solo adventure. In this scenario, the mother has a partner who is sensitive to her mood swings and is willing to listen and talk.

In the fight against postpartum depression, loved ones can be invaluable tools if you choose not to attribute the changes you've experienced to the typical challenges of parenthood. By working together, we can create an atmosphere that is welcoming and encouraging of help-seeking and the first steps on the road to recovery.

This chapter attempts to provide a nuanced understanding of postpartum depression by delving into real-life experiences and relevant instances. It is a call to action for moms, their loved ones, and healthcare providers to build an open, compassionate, and proactive attitude toward postpartum mental health treatments.

Chapter Five

Strategies and Methods for Developing

Resilience

My sleepy arms cuddled my fussy newborn in the dark of night as rains played a lullaby against the glass. In the midst of these private battles, when I felt the ebb and flow of mother anxieties, the idea of resilience became a lifeline, a slender but unyielding flame blazing in the darkness.

Constructing Resistance: Methods for

Withstanding Adversity

Resilience training is an art that requires a variety of techniques:

1.) Methods of Mindfulness: Mindfulness can be practised in short bursts throughout the day, for instance, during breastfeeding, by focusing on the physical sensation of breathing. In the midst of chaos, this routine serves to ground the mind.

2.) Methods of Self-Compassion: Shielding Against Self-Judgment Example: When faced with the unavoidable problems of motherhood, practice self-compassion by accepting faults without self-criticism. Be as compassionate with yourself as you would be with a friend who is going through a tough time.

3.) Create a list of positive affirmations that speak to you and repeat them often as an example. Statements such as, "I am strong and capable" When I overcome adversity, I become more powerful. The accumulation of such encouragement helps one develop a tough mentality.

4.) Example of setting healthy limits with family and friends in regards to visits and assistance: be open and honest about what you need from them. Establishing defined limitations protects mental and emotional well-being, ensuring a balanced attitude to parenthood.

5.) Preserving Daily Rituals for Added Stability. Example: Create daily routines that include both you and the baby. Stable routines give new mothers a sense of security that aids them as they face the unpredictability of postpartum difficulties.

(These aren't just words on paper; they're the instruments that kept us going through the restless nights.)

6.) Support from trained professionals: beacons in the night. Individual resilience suffers without the guidance of people who are familiar with the environment.

To further emphasise the significance of professional support in developing resilience, consider the following. Some details of this essential help are as follows:

Professional Advice: With the help of a professional, you can get advice that is specifically designed for your needs.

Emotional Compassion: Therapists and counsellors provide a safe place to talk about difficult feelings.

Healthcare providers create individualised plans to help new mothers and their families face the difficulties of the postpartum period.

Encouragement and affirmation: Acknowledging and supporting individuals through their difficulties helps them feel valued and motivated.

Chapter Six

Creating a Supportive Environment

When you become a mother, you quickly realize how important it is to have a strong support system. This chapter exposes an arsenal of tangible strategies and practical suggestions, giving a blueprint for establishing a resilient and supportive environment during the postpartum journey.

Creating a Comfortable Emotional Environment

1.) Encourage free and honest communication by creating a safe space for it. Share feelings, problems, and successes freely.

2.) Active and empathic listening within a support system is essential.

3.) Partners, family, and friends can help ease the emotional strain of caring for a newborn by taking on some of the day-to-day tasks involved.

4.) Adopt a collaborative strategy as a family. By working together, partners are better able to overcome obstacles and develop a mutual sense of responsibility and competence.

5.) In the midst of all the responsibilities of parenthood, it is important to make time for each other. This creates a chance to reconnect on an emotional level and offers respite.

6.) Facilitating Mutual Comprehension: Share your knowledge with your group to debunk myths and misconceptions regarding postpartum difficulties. Understanding and compassion are developed via learning.

7.) Community Engagement: Engage with local community groups or online forums to interact with other parents facing similar issues. The bond between people is strengthened by their shared history.

Wisdom from Grandma: A Solid Foundation

- Generational discussions: Facilitate discussions between generations, allowing for the exchange of wisdom and insights. Grandmothers have a wealth of knowledge to share with their grandchildren.

- Help Around the House and in the Kitchen Grandmothers may be a huge help around the house and in the kitchen, and they can even lend a hand when it comes to taking care of the infant.

Challenges of Cross-Cultural Communication

Engage in Free and frank discussion regarding your family's cultural norms and practices. Think about how you may strike a balance between these and your own wants and happiness.

Customizing Traditions: Modifying cultural practices to suit one's own ease and happiness. Change traditions to reflect the complexities of contemporary parenthood.

Advice from Experts in Other Fields than

Medicine

Doulas after Childbirth: Think about hiring a postpartum doula, a professional who helps new mothers with anything from practical tasks to emotional support and education.

Therapy and counseling can be a great source of further help when you're feeling down. Experts in mental health can advise and teach you how to use coping mechanisms.

Building a Community of Caring Support

Self-Care Education: Educate the support system on the value of self-care. To keep the support going strong, remind everyone to take care of themselves.

Help people learn to establish positive limits on their relationships with others in their support network. Clear boundaries create a sustainable and balanced approach.

Establishing Bonding Customs

Establishing a routine of eating together as a family can do wonders for bonding. Having dinner together is a great way to get to know one another and talk openly.

Intentional Moments: Plan get-togethers or special occasions with the people you care about, like dinner or a movie.

Independence's Long Road

Gradual Autonomy: Encourage autonomy gradually as resilience grows. Facilitate growth toward independence while sustaining social support.

To develop a sense of empowerment, encourage those involved in the support system to participate in decision-making and problem-solving.

Chapter Seven

Self-Care and Wellness Practices

The idea that parenthood is synonymous with self-neglect is a dissonance we attempt to dispel in this chapter. Instead, the importance of self-care only grows when you become a parent, because a well-cared-for caregiver is more likely to produce a healthy offspring. Give birth to the conviction that self-care after childbirth is not a sign of weakness but rather an invitation to rediscover a stronger, more confident you.

Moments of Reflection: Approach each new day with purpose and concentration. Take some deep breaths, meditate, or write down your ideas in a journal first thing in the morning when it's calm and peaceful. These interactions provide the groundwork for a day of intentional parenting.

Nourishing Nutrition: Reframe your approach to food as an expression of love for yourself. Prepare dishes that will satisfy your hunger and your taste buds. Taking care of yourself is a gift you can provide your child in the form of positive energy.

Constantly Refreshing Your Water Supply: Make drinking water into an elaborate ceremony. Use fresh fruit slices or aromatic herbs to flavor your water. Allow each sip to be a moment of revitalization that serves as a gentle reminder to feed your soul as well as your body.

Soothing Showers: Transform everyday showers into therapeutic rituals. Pick out some soothing music and a fragrant shower gel, and let the water wash away the mental tiredness that frequently comes along with being a new mom.

Happy Dance: View activity not as a task but as a celebration of your body's resiliency. Take your kid on slow strolls, do some yoga, or start dancing on the spot. Instead of viewing physical activity as a chore, try viewing it as a source of pleasure.

A good night's sleep is essential to your health, so make it a top priority. Create a calm pre-bedtime ritual, make your bedroom a restful place to be, and appreciate the rejuvenating effects of a good night's sleep.

Make room in your schedule for artistic pursuits that make you happy. Painting, writing, and other forms of creative expression provide a safe space to release tension, refuel, and rediscover who you are apart from your position as a parent.

Nature Connection: Wrap yourself in the loving arms of Mother Earth. Get out of the house and go for long walks in neighboring parks; the healing power of nature will do you good. Spending time in nature like this can do wonders for your mental health.

Support your social health by investing in your relationships with others. Plan consistent times to talk, whether that's through video chats or in-person get-togethers. The relationships you create outside of parenthood can become invaluable sources of strength.

Set aside times each week to unplug from electronics. Disconnect from screens, allowing your mind to unwind and reconnect with the analog world. Get back to basics and rediscover the pleasure of analog pursuits.

Mistreatment of Animals: Integrate pampering into your routine. Let the act of treating yourself, be it with expensive skin care products, spa days at home, or paid massages, be something to be celebrated.

Go on a reading retreat and lose yourself in the written word. Reading is a wonderful way to escape into another world of ideas and thoughts, whether it be a work of fiction, a self-help book, or a collection of poetry.

Laughter therapy emphasizes the use of humor for healing. Spend time doing things that make you happy, watch comedy, and put yourself in situations that will make you laugh.

Connecting the Mind and Body: Try doing some Tai Chi or some guided meditation. These methods promote health on all levels by strengthening the bond between the mind and body, which in turn improves physical health.

Engage in some learning excursions to get your brain working. Continuous learning, whether in the form of a new pastime, an online course, or the exploration of themes that tickle one's intellectual curiosity, leads to a feeling of development.

Rituals of Gratitude: Make being grateful part of your everyday routine. Keep a thankfulness notebook and take time to appreciate the many blessings in your life. Practicing gratitude often can be a great way to keep a happy outlook.

Therapeutic Touch: Incorporate therapeutic touch into your lifestyle. Touch becomes a language of self-care, promoting relaxation and stress alleviation, whether through self-massage, essential oil use, or professional treatments.

Use music as a therapeutic tool: This is "music medicine." Curate playlists that resonate with your emotions, attend live performances, and let the rhythm and song be a cure for your soul.

Boundary Establishment: Create safe zones around yourself to prevent harm. Master the art of assertive refusal, set boundaries, and cultivate an environment that supports your psychological and emotional well-being. Respecting oneself entails doing things like setting limits.

Write freely to better understand your feelings, obstacles, and successes. Writing in a journal can be a therapeutic way to explore your thoughts and feelings.

Chapter Eight

Overcoming Challenges and Obstacles

Obstacles and difficulties are constant companions on the transforming adventure that is parenthood. This chapter encourages you to shift your perspective from seeing obstacles as insurmountable hurdles to seeing them as stepping stones on the path to becoming a stronger, more confident parent. Use this inquiry as a map to navigate the challenges of motherhood, with the hope that you'll gain strength and wisdom from the experience.

In the world of parenting, there are no mistakes, only lovely details. Embrace the messy moments, realizing that growth often occurs from the midst of confusion.

Recognize the landscape of sleep deprivation, and learn to adapt to it. Find ways to get more sleep, such as taking naps when the baby does, splitting up nighttime responsibilities with a partner, or reaching out to friends and family for help.

Striking a balance between job and family life is like dancing on eggshells. To avoid burnout, it's important to set boundaries, express your requirements to your employer, and take care of yourself.

Relationship changes are inevitable after you become a parent. Spend some time talking things out, learning more about each other, and reaching out for help when you both need it. It's important to take care of your relationship even when you face obstacles as parents.

Although widespread, mother guilt presents a significant challenge for many people. You can be a better parent by taking care of yourself, which isn't selfish. Society puts a lot of pressure on parents to be perfect.

Parenthood can put a strain on one's bank account due to the higher costs associated with raising a family. Make a sensible spending plan, look at ways to cut costs, and get professional help if necessary.

The stability of a family depends on its members' ability to recognize and cope with financial stress.

Parenting has unique challenges when it comes to time management. Prioritize work, distribute duties, and realize the significance of self-care among a busy schedule. Time management skills help you live a life that's less chaotic and more satisfying.

Dealing with Unsolicited counsel Unsolicited counsel is a constant obstacle that many people face. Develop assertiveness in setting boundaries, gently ignoring unsolicited counsel, and following your instincts as a parent.

Postpartum depression is a serious problem that needs to be addressed as part of postpartum care. To deal with the challenges of postpartum mental health, it's important to get treatment from professionals, surround yourself with caring people, and put your own needs first.

Partners often have different parenting philosophies from one another. Make an effort to talk things out, agree on some things, and raise your kids as a team. Parenting is easier when both parents can listen to and value each child's ideas and feelings.

Confronting Health Problems You Didn't See Coming: Facing unexpected health problems can be nerve-wracking. If you're worried about your health, it's important to see a doctor often, learn about preventative measures, and get advice from experts.

Sibling interactions provide an additional layer of complication that must be navigated. Create a welcoming atmosphere, promote open lines of communication, and find productive solutions to any issues that arise. Fostering close relationships between siblings helps keep the peace at home.

Maintaining a healthy sense of who you are as an individual while still fulfilling your role as a parent is a continuous challenge. Focus on developing your own interests and passions alongside your parental duties.

Challenges in parenting arise while dealing with children that exhibit challenging behaviors. Approach behavioral challenges with compassion, consistency, and empathy; seek support from parenting resources; if required, seek professional advice.

Being a parent requires you to be adaptable, as plans are constantly changing. Develop your capacity to roll with the punches, expect the unexpected, and see change not as a threat but as an opportunity.

Concerns about children's education are natural and should be addressed as they develop. Participate in your child's education by learning about and discussing alternatives with teachers.

Dealing with Peer Pressure: Dealing with social demands can be intimidating. Put in place limits, make the well-being of your family a top priority, and center your attention on ideals that reflect your parenting stance.

Dealing with Loss and Grief: As a parent, you may experience loss and grief. Get the help you need emotionally, try some therapeutic activities, and give yourself some space and time to work through these difficult feelings.

The only constant in parenthood is change. Appreciate the beauty in the process as you and your loved ones adapt to the ever-changing world around you.

Most importantly, train yourself to be resilient. The ups and downs of parenting are like a complicated dance. Strengthen your ability to recover quickly from challenges, grow as a parent as a result of your

experiences, and overcome adversity.

Chapter Nine

Celebrating Progress and Milestones

As we begin this new phase, I'd want to invite you to join me in honoring the development, resiliency, and love that have emerged as a result of your efforts as a parent. It's a chance to take stock of what's been accomplished, celebrate the good times, and look forward with excitement to the wonderful new chapters that lie ahead.

Historic Firsts: Relish the magical "firsts" that mark your journey as a parent, from the first grin to the first steps. Every achievement is a tribute to your parenting skills and a symbol of your child's maturation.

Recognizing Developmental Changes: Being a parent is a life-changing event for both you and your kid. Think about how you've changed as a person, the skills you've developed, and the tenacity that's come to define you.

Establishing rituals in honor of significant life events fosters a feeling of continuity and camaraderie. Whether it's a special family dinner, a photo shoot, or a loving letter to your child, these rituals give depth to the significance of each milestone.

In the hectic pace of parenthood, remember to pause and record those fleeting, unforgettable moments. Take pictures, make a movie, or keep a journal to look back on and remember the amazing memories you've made together.

Share the joy of success with your loved ones. Make it a point to recognize and applaud everyone's successes, no matter how modest. Your optimism will serve as the engine that drives your success.

Expectation Management Celebrate by setting realistic expectations. Every stage of parenthood has its ups and downs, and not every achievement deserves a celebration. Small successes can have a profound impact on one's outlook.

Expressing Gratitude: Gratitude multiplies the delight of milestones. Appreciate your child's existence, development, and individuality by pausing to give thanks. Having a heart full of gratitude will improve your parenting.

Establishing New Customs as a Family: Creating new rituals to celebrate significant life events bonds families together. Every family has its own set of traditions, whether it's an annual trip, a holiday feast, or something else entirely.

Dealing Effectively with Adversity: To appreciate success is not to ignore failure; rather, it is to master the art of dealing with both. Recognize difficulties, gain wisdom from them, and look for opportunities in adversity.

Recognizing and Celebrating Differences: Your parenting experience will be as unique as your child. Honor the unique route your family is forging and the uniqueness of your child. Acceptance and love may flourish when people embrace their individuality.

Making a Milestone Timeline Draw up a milestone timeline to help you picture the development process. This timeline, whether printed out or kept digitally, will evolve to reflect the significant milestones in your parenting journey.

Celebrating Parenting achievements: As a parent, notice and celebrate your personal achievements. Everything you do as a parent, no matter how big or tiny, has an impact on your family.

Training Your Brain for Success: Embrace a growth mindset as you celebrate progress. Appreciate the ever-changing nature of your family and view setbacks as opportunities to learn and grow together.

Extend the party by telling others you care about about your accomplishments. Whether through phone conversations, text messages, or in-person get-togethers, include your loved ones increases the joy and improves your network of friends and family.

Contemplation of Adversity Conquered: Give some thought to the difficulties you've conquered. Honor not only your successes, but also your ability to overcome adversity and move forward. Your perseverance thus far is an inspiration.

Fostering Autonomy Major life events can represent turning points on the path to autonomy. Celebrating and encouraging your child's growing feeling of autonomy might help them develop a strong sense of self.

Parenthood is a lifelong learning experience, and that fact deserves to be celebrated. Acknowledging that development is a never-ending, ever-changing process, you and your child should relish each and every teaching opportunity.

Embrace the principles that make your family unique and celebrate major life events in ways that reflect those ideals. Anchoring celebrations in these principles, whether it's love, kindness, or perseverance, lends depth and significance to the festivities.

Planning for Future Milestones: Anticipation of future milestones adds an exciting aspect to your journey. Think ahead and make plans for future successes to be honored.

Take a minute to reflect on the full journey as you enjoy the successes along the way. Parenthood is a complicated, ever-evolving tapestry that incorporates every stride, every stumble, and every accomplishment.

In celebrating accomplishments and milestones, remember that the trip is as significant as the destination. You've handled the curveballs thrown at you with grace and affection. I hope this new chapter in your life serves as a source of inspiration for you and your family as you continue to grow as parents and as individuals.

I did it and so can you. You really can. Go Mom!